MW01290633

THE KETOGENIC DIET FOR BEGINNERS

Table of Contents

INTRODUCTION: WHAT ARE KETOGENIC DIETS?

Dr. Russell Wilder, a physician from the infamous Mayo Clinic, designed the ketogenic diet in 1928 with the primary intention of creating a food based cure for epilepsy. It was highly successful, but unfortunately the diet itself was discarded with the inception of anti-seizure drugs in the 1940's. However, studies show that ketogenic diets are an effective way to combat seizures when medication is no longer an option.

The idea of these types of diets are simply to restrict carbohydrate intake, and to control the glucose concentration in the blood. A normal body uses mostly carbohydrates to provide the energy needs; carbohydrates are converted to glucose that is then oxidized in the body's cells to provide energy for it to function.

In the event the body has low carbohydrate levels, our bodies are forced to find other sources of energy, usually resulting in the burning of fat through a process called 'ketosis'. During ketosis, fats are broken down in the liver into fatty acids and ketone bodies. The ketone bodies are then oxidized to provide energy, replacing carbohydrates, as the main energy source that our bodies use to function.

As you can see, ketogenic diets don't just fight against epilepsy; they are a very effective way of getting both blood sugar and weight under control, forcing the body to use stored fat to power itself through daily activities.

This book will cover how the diet works, what the body does when it's in a state of ketosis, recipes for ketosis friendly foods, and a sample meal plan to get you started. Whether you are looking to start this type of diet as a response to epilepsy related issues or simply to lose weight, it's our hope that this title will be a good starting point to getting your body and life back in control.

ABOUT KETOSIS

Ketosis isn't just a process, it's a 'state' that reflects how exactly the body is generating it's energy. This condition is marked by higher than normal ketone levels in the blood and occurs when the body does not have enough glucose (from carbohydrates) to burn for energy. Because Ketosis is really the body burning fat for energy for various body metabolisms, it's common in thoughts that have experienced starvation or are on some sort of fast. While it sounds serious there really is no reason for alarm if the body is in a 'ketosis' state as it is a very normal process. There is, however, usually a period of adjustment (usually less than a week) where the body gets used to using fats as its main energy source.

KETOACIDOSIS

Ketoacidosis is a metabolic state associated with very high levels of keton bodies. There keton bodies are formed from the breakdown of fats and the deamination of proteins. It is marked by extreme and uncontrolled ketosis and in this state, the body fails to regulate ketone production which results in a buildup of keto acids. These acids decreases the blood pH, and in instances of prolonged ketosis, it can be fatal if not monitored.

Diabetic Ketoacidosis

A serious complication occurs when the body produces high levels of ketons due to insufficient insulin. Normally glucose, which is a major energy source in the bloodstream, enters into the cells with the help of insulin that our bodies produce. Because the pancreas produces insulin, its failure means little or no insulin is produced and puts the body in to a diabetic state. This will result into a buildup of glucose in the blood stream, causing high blood sugar levels, and because the body is deprived of its energy source it breaks down fat to produce ketones. This increased sugar in the blood stream overloads the kidneys, and as a result the kidneys respond by pushing additional glucose in our urine to expel it from the body. The result is dehydration as water moves from blood to urine by osmosis and if untreated, can be fatal.

Alcoholic Ketoacidosis

Alcohol causes dehydration in the body and can hinder the first step of gluconeogenesis, or the body's ability to generate enough glucose to meet its needs. This depletion of energy providing nutrients will cause the body to break down body fat to produce ketones, much like starvation, but with the access sugar provided from alcohol. Alcohol can inhibit the ability of the pancreas to produce insulin as well, which means that the glucose would not be absorbed to body cells, which can cause the body to produce ketones. This will cause a buildup of ketones in the bloodstream leading to the case of acidosis.

Causes of Ketoacidosis

Insulin deficiency

Insulin is primarily responsible for how glucose is absorbed into body cells, which is later used as energy. Depletion of insulin causes the body to be deprived of glucose, forcing it to breakdown fats to produce ketones. Some underlying factors can cause insulin deficiency

1. **An underlying infection**

   The body's response to an infection is to produce more glucose so that it can provide energy for disease fighting cells, and these glucose levels may be generated in excess compared to the amount of insulin being produced. This means less glucose will be processed and the body may turn it to fat to later be used for energy. The most common infections include:

- Pneumonia

- Influenza(flu)

- Gastroenteritis- an infection of the digestive system

- Urinary Tract Infection (UTI) – This is an infection of the urinary tract and the bladder.

2. Missed Treatment

Some patients, especially those that are diabetic, may at times miss important treatments such as insulin injections. This may aggravate the body as it becomes more and more deprived of glucose, resulting in converting the bodily fat into ketones.

3. Undiagnosed Diabetes

If someone has Type 1 Diabetes and it is undiagnosed, this disease can develop quickly into diabetic ketoacidosis. Therefore, it is extremely important for people visit their physician at the slightest sign of Type 1 Diabetes.

4. Drinking a lot of Alcohol

Large amounts of alcohol can hinder the body from producing a healthy amount of glucose and inhibit the production of insulin. This is very important to ensure the regulation of glucose in the blood. If not kept in check, then it can lead to a severe case of alcoholic ketoacidosis.

SIGNS THAT YOU ARE IN KETOSIS

Signs and symptoms of ketosis can start to appear in as early as a week, but for some people (like professional athletes), it may take as long as 12 weeks to notice any effect. Here are some of the signs that point to ketosis:

❖ **Bad breath**

This is usually a very common sign of low carb ketosis. One may notice a particular 'fruity' smell in their breath. This is usually acetone, which is a byproduct of the ketosis process that is released in our breath. Bad breath can also be caused by dehydration, so it is advisable to drink a lot of water to reduce the concentration of ketons in your body.

❖ **Reduced appetite and Increased Thirst**

Many people in low carb ketosis diet have reported a lack of appetite as they reach ketosis. Nausea, one of the side effects of ketosis, can also reduce your appetite for food. Your lack of appetite may also be due to an increased intake of proteins, and in addition, increased concentration of ketones causes a diuretic effect. This means that the body is prone to dehydration, which makes it paramount to drink additional water to avoid dehydration.

❖ **Urine Test**

As the body burns fat, it produces ketones. Acetone is a byproduct ketone that the body is unable to use produce energy. Because of this, the body disposes it as waste through urine and the moisture in our breath.

One of the ways to test for ketosis is by using ketone test strips. These strips measure the amount of ketones in your urine to find out if you are positive for ketosis. It's important to remember, however, that the results can be influenced by the amount of water you drink. For instance, if you drink a lot of water then it may dilute the ketones in the urine and may result in a negative test even though your body may be in a state of ketosis.

❖ Increased Energy

You are likely to start feeling more energetic when your body adjusts to a low carb diet. When the body breaks down fat and the ketones are oxidized, they produce a higher amount of energy than for the same equal amount of glucose. Because more energy is released for a unit of fat burned, most people are likely to experience increased energy levels. This is why many professional athletes prefer a kategonic diet since it provides them with more energy to do energy intensive trainings and sports.

❖ Feelings of Wellbeing or Euphoria

The brain prefers to use ketones as its main energy source because it yields more energy per unit burned. Because the brain has more energy than it is used to working with, it may trigger feelings of euphoria and a general sense of well being.

❖ Mental Clarity

This is experienced by those people who have seizures and epilepsy. With the increased levels of ketones in the blood stream, the frequencies of epileptic seizures are significantly reduced which may make you feel mentally clear.

❖ Ketosis Flu

This is one of the side effects that many people experience when they switch to a low carb diet. It is also known as the induction flu and usually marks the transition period when the body starts to use ketones instead of glucose. Its symptoms include:

- Nausea

- Headaches

- Stomach Upsets

- Fatigue

- Lack of Mental Clarity

- Sleepiness

This usually happens within the first few days when the ketogenic diet starts and is perfectly normal.

ADVANTAGES OF A KETOGENIC DIET

Being in a ketosis state has many advantages, some of which can even be life saving in some circumstances. Below are some of the benefits you get when on a low carb diet:

1. One of the main advantages of this diet is that it forces the body to utilize body fat for fuel. If you are on a carbohydrate friendly diet, the body breaks it down into glucose as the body prefers to oxidize glucose rather than body fat. Ketosis makes the body efficient in burning bodily fat which many people find pleasurable as this results in significant weight loss.

2. When the body has no use for excess ketones, it will simply excrete them out mainly as urine. This is in contrast to a high carb diet where excess glucose is converted into fat for later use. A low carb diet does not only make us lose body fat, but also maintain body shape as no fat deposits are made.

3. In ketosis, protein in the body is spared from oxidation to glucose through glucenogenesis. In this state, the body actually prefers ketones to glucose because it has vast reserves of bodily fat. Because of the fat stores, there is no need to oxidize proteins meaning one only needs to eat an adequate amount of proteins.

4. Having a ketogenic diet helps lower your insulin levels because insulin has the ability to prevent the conversion of fat to energy. Normal diets make for high levels of insulin that inhibits lypolysis. Lowered insulin levels will increase lipolysis, causing more fat to be burned. In addition, the lowered insulin levels allows for the

release of other beneficial hormones to keep the body at it's best.

5. Ketone bodies are very inefficient fuel. This means that they have very little calories relative to their mass, therefore, if the body is in ketosis, it will burn a lot of fat but will not produce as many calories. If your goal is to lose a lot of weight, ketosis will be able to trim you back to shape in a short time.

6. The majority of the fat that is burned is from the abdominal cavity. Not all fat is the same; we have the subcantenous fat and visceral fat. Subcantenous fat is lodged underneath the skin and helps us to stay warm. Visceral fat, however, is the fat that forms around organs (usually in the abdominal cavity) that can drive inflammation, insulin resistance, and cause metabolic dysfunction. This visceral fat is burned during ketosis, getting rid of belly fat.

7. Ketosis reduces blood sugar and insulin levels. When we eat high carb diets, the sugar is broken down into glucose in the digestive tract where it is absorbed into the bloodstream. When it enters the blood stream, it causes a spike in blood sugar. Healthy people will produce insulin that will regulate the sugar levels, but some people have insulin resistance and are unable to regulate blood sugar levels that might lead to type 2 diabetes. Ketosis arrests this situation by lowering the amount of available glucose in the blood, thus reducing the need for insulin.

8. Ketosis helps treat a number of brain disorders. Some parts of the brain can only use glucose, but the majority can also use ketones when carbohydrate intake is very

low. The ketogenic diet was originally developed for epileptic seizures and has helped many with that condition because of this. Some studies have shown over half of patients on a ketogenic diet had a 50% reduction in seizures, and others made a full recovery.

9. People can lose weight on a ketogenic diet. A lot of unwanted body weight is due to fat reserves deposited in the body and ketosis serves to lower carbohydrate intake, forcing your body to burn fat to produce energy. Due to the inefficiency of fat as a fuel, a lot of it has to be burned to release a relatively small amount of energy. Thus, ketosis can be very helpful in shedding that extra weight. There have been reported cases where people have lost up to 160 pounds by simply using ketogenic diets.

DISADVANTAGES OF THE KETOGENIC DIET

Although ketosis comes with many advantages, it has some disadvantages as well. Obviously, the advantages outweigh the disadvantages by a huge margin, but you should still watch out for some of these drawbacks.

1. Your body has to undergo a transition stage as your body adjusts to using ketones. During this transition period you may experience a number of side effects including fatigue, headaches, and nausea. The good news is that it is very short lived, so you can expect to go back to normalcy within a short amount of time.

2. Since the ketogenic diet requires an increased intake of fats, it can cause the blood lipids to increase. This means instead of reducing cholesterol in the blood stream, the high intake of fats can cause the reverse effect of increasing cholesterol levels.

3. Because foods rich in carbohydrates are restricted, you can have a deficiency of micronutrients that accompany those foods. This may lead to deficiency related conditions or diseases, so the best way to tackle this situation is by making sure you take vitamin and mineral supplements. Additionally, remember to consume a lot of fiber to aid in digestion.

4. Ketoacidosis can also be a disadvantage of a ketogenic diet. This is because the ketone levels in your blood stream can spike and get out of control and this can lead to acidosis. This lowers the blood PH and can be fatal if not treated. This cannot affect non-diabetic

people as their bodies keep blood sugar low and allow only 'just enough ketones' to be produced at any one time.

MOTIVATION TO CHANGE

Motivating yourself can be a challenge. It's not that you don't want to loose weight, of course you do, but there is a lot of work between where you are now and where you want to be. It can feel helpless and be incredibly difficult to stay motivated; and one candy bar won't mess everything up, right?

The Right Frame of Mind

This diet will only work if you are in the right frame of mind and continuously motivate and encourage yourself to make the right exercise and eating choices every time. It's easy to make the right decisions when it's, well, easy, but what do you do when you are at that holiday party? Or late at night when you're starving and all you want is cookies?

Just Start

It's never a perfect time to start dieting. Life will always be stressful, there will always be a holiday coming up, or some event that will make it difficult for you to stay on board. Just pick a day, dedicate yourself to starting on that day, and just do it.

It's Really Not a Choice

Logic dictates that if you aren't at a healthy weight or don't care of your body, there will be consequences. It might not be now, but it will happen eventually and this could affect your spouse, children, work, and family. You owe it to yourself and the people important to you to take care of yourself to ensure you live a long healthy life with the people you love. You can keep eating and living life the way you do, but if you want to continue to be there for those around you, you don't have any choice but to change.

Make Smaller Goals

If you have 100 pounds to loose, and you focus on that number, you may feel like you are fighting a loosing battle. Break your big goal up in to smaller, more manageable pieces. If you plan to loose 100 pounds and want to do it in a year and a half, think of your 'mini' goals as 5 pounds a month, or better yet 1 to 2 pounds a week. This gives you something to focus on, something easy and close to achieve. Before you know it, three months later, you've lost almost 20 pounds and it didn't feel like the most mentally exhausting thing you've ever done.

Chart It

Record your successes and failures. If you keep a list of where you went wrong, you'll know what to avoid later. If you had a good week, think over why it was so successful and try and recreate it in the weeks to come. By charting your diet, you can generate momentum and help motivate yourself to keep at it.

Stay Positive

Remind yourself of everything positive that's happening around you. You are making a difference, you've decided to make a major change in your life. This is a good thing! So you don't want to have a giant piece of chocolate cake, and that's sad. But, you do love the way that peach smoothie tastes first thing in the morning, and that's something that makes you feel good without messing up your dieting plan. Enjoy that peach smoothie and try to distract yourself from the chocolate cake. Trying to stay positive will help keep you in the right frame of mind.

REWARD YOURSELF

If you've done good, reward yourself with some frozen yogurt or a trip to the movies. Buy a new pair of jeans when you've hit a weight milestone. These rewards not only make you feel good, but they fuel you to keep going when your 'dieting tank' is low.

Determine why you want to lose weight

If you really don't have something to justify your inner drive, the diet likely won't be successful. Your reasons could include being healthy, to look good in a bikini, or to have more energy. Whatever your motivation, you should know it to ensure that it keeps you focused on your goal. Find a way of keeping the pressure on by ensuring that you are constantly reminded of what it is you want to achieve; try hanging a picture on your bathroom mirror to remind you or hang a motivation poster in your kitchen. The diet itself will just be a journey that helps you get to your goals!

Make yourself accountable

Simply having to talk to someone else about the diet will provide just the right amount of pressure to deter you in some situations. If you cannot find anyone to be accountable to, be accountable to yourself. You may want to use special habit building apps or simply record your weight regularly to see how well you are doing. If you have to weigh yourself, do it over a span of a week; doing it daily could be frustrating, especially if your weight seems to fluctuate.

How To Set Goals

There is an art form to goal setting; it takes skill to figure out what you want and how to get there and it's important to do just that when you are setting goals for yourself.

Start with the End

In the beginning, it's good to know what the ultimate goal is and what exactly you are striving for. If you want to loose 100 pounds at the end of this dieting endeavor, then that is your overall goal. If you want to move down 4 pant sizes, than this is what you should be striving for and all goals related to the diet and exercise should help you get there.

Make a list and break it up

When you know what your long term plan is, make a list of the things you will have to do to achieve this goal. Plan out how you will exercise, get together meal plans, and make sure you clearly understand what is involved in achieving this goal. When you write out your goals, write them as positive attainable statements. If you write them in a positive way, they'll make you feel positive and motivated about the goals you have set before you.

Take the list you made and break it up in to manageable sections. Categorize your mini goals about food and exercise in to groups that have to do with each other.

Prioritize and organize

Take the groups you made and rate them by order of importance, then break those further down in to chronological time frames. This will help you to stay focused and organized so you don't get side tracked during the dieting process. The more clear and obvious you make it for yourself, the easier it will be to reach your weight loss goals.

WHAT TO EAT ON A KETOGENIC DIET

There are different classes of foods that create the bulk of the Ketogenic Diet. It's important that these food classifications be consumed in the right amounts to achieve the benefits of a ketogenic diet.

ON 'NET CARBS'

As the popularity of 'low carb' diets has increased over the years, the question many health professionals are asking is, 'When is a carb not a carb?'

Food manufacturers want their customers to keep purchasing from them, so in an attempt to offer all of those tasty carb filled foods to low carb conscious dieters, a new category of carbohydrates was created. This new type of carbohydrate claims to offer all of the perks of carbohydrate foods without the down side.

The idea of 'net carbs' was founded in that not all carbohydrates work inside the body the same way. Some are absorbed quickly, forcing a spike in blood sugar levels. Others are stored as fat on the body for later use, and even some carbs (like fiber) work slowly through the digestive track with little of the food actually being absorbed.

Food manufacturers adjust their labels to sport the 'net carbs' on their products, which is almost always significantly less than what the foods actual food label reads. The important thing to note here is that anything on a FDA approved food label is reviewed and given clearance by the FDA, but manufacturers are still legally allowed to put misleading information on the front of the food labeling.

To calculate net carbs, food manufacturers take the total number of carbohydrates and subtract fiber and sugar alcohols. Why? The answer is simple; these carbohydrates are claimed to have little effect on blood sugar levels. Some physicians, however, warn that not all fiber and sugar alcohols work this way. In fact, in addition to having a laxative effect and adding calories to an already watched diet, some sugar alcohols can indeed raise blood sugar levels despite claims on the packaging.

FATS AND OILS

There has been a misinterpretation of fats over the years and people have even gone to extreme lengths to avoid fats all together. However, the main focus of the ketogenic diet is to provide the body with fats to be broken down to produce energy. It's for this reason that there is a heavy emphasis on the intake of fats and oils to provide the body with this type of fuel source. It's also important to remember that there are different types of fats; some can be good while others can be a health risk.

Saturated Fats

Saturated Fats keep your immunities at optimum levels, bone density normal, and testosterone levels in check. For a long time, these types of fats were categorized as one of the bad "trans-fats" that you shouldn't consume regularly. However, research has shown that they are very necessary for our health; in fact, they pose no risk to the overall health of the body. Foods that contain this type of fat include meat, eggs, and butter which help improve HDL/LDL cholesterol levels.

Polyunsaturated Fat

Polyunsaturated fats are highly processed and bad for your health. Studies have shown that cause of the majority of the heart diseases epidemic is due to liquid vegetable oil and trans-fats. For example, most of the margarines we spread on bread have these processed vegetable oils, so it may be a good idea to regulate its intake.

People should not be confused between natural polyunsaturated fat and processed polyunsaturated fat. Natural polyunsaturated fat, mostly found in fatty fish, help in improving HDL/LDL cholesterol levels. Processed polyunsaturated fat on the other hand ,worsens HDL/LDL cholesterol levels and therefore becomes risky to your health.

Monosaturated Fats

Olive and sunflower oils are some of the examples in this category. This type of fat has come to be widely accepted as healthy. Research has shown that they lead to better insulin resistance levels and better HDL/LDL cholesterol levels, which are beneficial to our overall health.

Trans Fats

Trans fats are not included in the category of fatty oils, but are worth mentioning as these fats result from chemical modification. The fats go through a hydrogenation process to improve their self-life, where the process adjusts the position of hydrogen in the fat molecule. This has been proven to be very harmful for our bodies. It can lead to higher HDL/LDL cholesterol levels that may pose great danger to your health.

Cholesterols and Fats

Cholesterol is a compound found in most body tissues. It is a very important constituent of cell membranes; these fats are constantly moving throughout your blood stream and danger arises when cholesterol particles bump into each other, forming lumps in major arteries. This can lead to a condition known as atherosclerosis, or the blockage of arteries that can lead to serious health risks such as heart attacks.

In addition to fats, HDL, LDL and triglycerides are also important to the make up of the body.

- HDL

    These are high-density lipoproteins. They are usually referred to as the 'good cholesterol' and are responsible for transferring cholesterol from body tissues to the liver to be broken down. They also help reduce the amount of LDL in the blood stream by removing unwanted cholesterol from the body's tissues and reducing the risk of vessel blockages and heart disease.

- LDL

    These are the low-density lipoproteins. This is the bad version of cholesterol. LDL takes processed cholesterol from the liver and transfers it into body tissues increasing the amount of cholesterol in the blood stream and the likelihood of developing arteriosclerosis and heart disease.

- Triglycerides

    When one consumes fatty foods, the fats are digested and absorbed into the tissues. While in the tissues, the fat takes the form of triglycerides to make it easy to transport between tissues and the blood stream.

Having a low LDL count reduces the chances of cholesterol particles bumping into each other and will reduce the risk of developing blockages. High triglyceride levels may need an increase in LDL so that they can be transported; this can increase the risk of clumping and increasing chances of a heart disease.

For ketogenic diets, you should consume foods rich in omega 3 fatty oils, like salmon, tuna, and trout just to mention a few. Additionally, take saturated and monosaturated fats like butter, macadamia nuts, avocados, egg yolks, and coconut oils. These are preferred because they have a stable chemical structure, which is less inflammatory to the body.

You should aim to reduce your trans-fat intake. This means avoiding use of hydrogenated fats, as they have a high trans-fat concentration that is bad for your health. In short, if you like fried foods, go for non-hydrogenated options like ghee and coconut oil. This ensures that oxidation of these oils is at a minimum, which means you will get the essential oils without all the trans-fat.

Be wary of the inflammatory omega 6 fatty oils. This can involve watching your intake of anything nut or seed based. Here is a list of ketogenic diet foods that are a great source of fat and oils that won't give you problems later:

- Avocado

- Butter

- Coconut oil

- Olive oil

- Chicken fat

- Peanut butter

- Non hydrogenated lard

PROTEINS

Proteins are responsible for the repair of worn out cells as well as general growth. Many of our body tissues are mostly protein; from our skin to our hair and even our nails. Proteins help in the creation and regulations of hormones in the blood stream that control various bodily functions.

In a ketogenic diet though, protein intake should be adequate. It should be just enough to satisfy your protein requirements and a high intake of proteins in a ketogenic diet may result to the body breaking down proteins for energy. This means the body will disintegrate its own tissues, and in the process, wear itself out.

There are various sources for protein for a ketogenic diet, which include:

- Fish of any type.

- White and Red Meat

Other sources can include shellfish like oysters, lobster, and crab. Whole eggs, bacon, and sausages also act as very good sources of proteins as well.

VEGTABLES

Vegetables are extremely important in a ketogenic diet. They are a huge source of vitamins which are required to generate and maintain a healthy immune system to fight diseases. Go for anything that is grown above ground and is leafy green. However, some vegetables are high in sugar and shouldn't be used in ketogenic diets. The best types of vegetables for this diet are high in nutrients, low on carbohydrates, and are usually dark and leafy. They include spinach and kales or any other vegetable that resembles them. The following can serve as good vegetables for a ketogenic diet:

- Spinach

- Broccoli

- Green beans

- Cucumbers

- Mushrooms

- Butterhead lettuce

- Pickles

- Cauliflowcr

- Asparagus

In addition, onions, tomatoes, and garlic can be included in a ketogenic diet.

DAIRY

Other things that should be incorporated into low carb diets include full fat dairy products. These include heavy whipped cream, hard and soft cheeses, sour cream, and cottage cheese.

BEVERAGES

One of the effects of having a ketogenic diet is that you will get very dehydrated so it is extremely important that you drink plenty of water in addition to other liquids like coffee and tea. Be careful not to drink any liquids that contain sugar as these will compromise your diet; staying away from sugary beverages is the best bet. If you crave for something sweet, it's okay to use liquid artificial sweeteners. Examples of sweeteners include:

- Stevia

- Suclarose

- Erythritol

- Xylitol

- Monk fruit

SPICES

Be very careful about the spices you use in your foods. Some spices are high in carbs because they are mostly premixed with sugars; even the common table salt is usually mixed with powdered dextrose, so many people consider using sea salt. Here is a list of spices that are good for low carb diets:

- Sea salt

- Black pepper

- Cinnamon

- Chili powder

- Turmeric

- Parsley

- Rosemary

- Sage

WHAT TO AVOID IN A KETOGENIC DIET

What exactly are foods that you should avoid on the ketogenic diet? The following can serve as a general list:

- Sugars: Avoid anything that has brown sugar, cane sugar, corn syrup, honey, or sucrose. In additional, avoid fruits as most have high levels of fructose and sucrose. In short, if it's 'sweet', don't eat it.

- Grain: This includes wheat, rice, sorghum, and barley and products made from these grains such as wheat flour, pasta, pancakes, cookies, and cakes.

- Corn: Avoid corn products like cornbread, corn chips, popcorn, and cornmeal. Corn can be used as a thickener or preservative in other products so remember to read labels.

- Starches: Avoid foods like potatoes, sweet potatoes, and yams. This also applies to their products such as potato chips, French fries, and tater tots.

- Boxed Processed Foods: Most of these foods are high in wheat and sugars and have high levels of carbs. In addition, avoid canned soups and stews as most contain hidden starchy thickeners.

- Fruits: Fruits of any kind are high in fructose. Berries have the lowest carbs; therefore, if you want to include a fruit in your diet, one or two berries will not hurt.

- Legumes: This includes beans, peanuts, and lentils that have very high starch content.

- Beer: Beers are a product of grain, which has high carb content. If you have to drink, consume low carb beers.

- Non Diet Sodas: Sweetened soda contains large amounts of fructose and corn syrup, which has lots of carbs that you should avoid.

- Milk: Especially skimmed milk because it contains a type of sugar known as lactose. Fermented milk products like yoghurt have less lactose because the bacteria used to ferment uses up all the lactose. If you have to include dairy, choose fermented products like these.

If you are planning to start a ketogenic diet you should plan to make many sacrifices, especially if you are a food lover. Cutting down on your sugar intake and avoiding starchy foods will go a long way to make the diet a success.

4 WEEK SAMPLE MEAL PLAN

WEEK 1: Day 1

Breakfast: Eggs, Bacon

Lunch: Low carb pizza, Crispy green beans

Dinner: Asian pork chops with some steamed cauliflower

WEEK 1: Day 2

Breakfast: Eggs, Sausage

Lunch: Spinach Salad

Dinner: Bacon Wrapped Chicken Breast and steamed broccoli

WEEK 1: Day 3

Breakfast: Low carb beacon frittata

Lunch: Low carb chili con carne

Dinner: Cauliflower fried rice and Butter paneer chicken cur

WEEK 1: Day 4

Breakfast: Blueberry Lemon Muffins

Lunch: Basil Pesto

Dinner: Meatloaf

WEEK 1: Day 5

Breakfast: Cheese Muffins

Lunch: Baked Salmon and Steam Broccoli

Dinner: Steamed yellow squash with basil, and Chicken with Herbed Cream Sauce

WEEK 1: Day 6

Breakfast: Cheese Muffins

Lunch: Spinach Salad with Grilled Chicken Breast

Dinner: Herb Baked Salmon and Grilled Asparagus

WEEK 1: Day 7

Breakfast: Pancakes*

Lunch: Keto Pizza Bites*

Dinner: Parmesan Crusted Pork Loin*

WEEK 2: Day 1

Breakfast: Trail Mix Cereal*

Lunch: Breadless Italian 'Sub'*

Dinner: Low Carb Meatballs*

WEEK 2: Day 2

Breakfast: Pumpkin Cream cheese Pancakes*

Lunch: Squash Noodle Lo Mein*

Dinner: Apple Cider Brussel Sprout Salad* and Grilled Salmon

WEEK 2: Day 3

Breakfast: Keto Cereal*

Lunch: Egg Drop Soup*

Dinner: Chili Con Queso**

WEEK 2: Day 4

Breakfast: Cheese Muffins

Lunch: Buffalo Pulled Chicken*

Dinner: Spiced Moroccan Stuffed Peppers***

WEEK 2: Day 5

Breakfast: Eggs, Bacon

Lunch: Garlic Cauliflower Breadsticks*

Dinner: Low Carb Pizza with Cauliflower Crust*

WEEK 2: Day 6

Breakfast: Eggs, Sausage

Lunch: Buffalo Wings*

Dinner: Lemon Cream Chicken over Squash Pasta*

WEEK 2: Day 7

Breakfast: Pancakes*

Lunch: Roast Beef Breadless Sandwich*

Dinner: Chicken Ranch Bacon Tacos*

WEEK 3: Day 1

Breakfast: Blueberry Lemon Muffins

Lunch: Chicken Soup*

Dinner: Steak and Pastrami Bomb*

WEEK 3: Day 2

Breakfast: Baked Eggs with Avocados***

Lunch: Lemon Garlic Keto Pasta*

Dinner: Chicken and Pancetta*

WEEK 3: Day 3

Breakfast: Eggie Cups **

Lunch: Philly Cheese Steak Stuffed Peppers*

Dinner: Spaghetti Squash Lasagna*

WEEK 3: Day 4

Breakfast: Low carb beacon frittata

Lunch: Low carb pizza, Crispy green beans

Dinner: Crispy Lemon and Thyme Stuffed Chicken Thighs*

WEEK 3: Day 5

Breakfast: Blueberry Lemon Muffins

Lunch: Spinach Salad

Dinner: Beanless Keto Chili*

WEEK 3: Day 6

Breakfast: Eggs, Bacon

Lunch: Keto Pizza Bites*

Dinner: Apple Cider Brussel Sprout Salad* and Grilled Salmon

WEEK 3: Day 7

Breakfast: Eggs, Sausage

Lunch: Low Carb Meatballs*

Dinner: Steak and Pastrami Bomb*

WEEK 4: Day 1

Breakfast: Spinach and Cheese Egg Bake**

Lunch: 'Everything in the Fridge' Salad**

Dinner: Parmesan Crusted Pork Loin*

WEEK 4: Day 2

Breakfast: Cheese Muffins

Lunch: Spinach Salad with Grilled Chicken Breast

Dinner: Low Carb Pizza with Cauliflower Crust*

WEEK 4: Day 3

Breakfast: Spinach and Cheese Quiche***

Lunch: Keto Pizza Bites*

Dinner: Herb Baked Salmon and Grilled Asparagus

WEEK 4: Day 4

Breakfast: Baked Eggs with Avocados***

Lunch: Loaded Roasted Califlower Soup***

Dinner: Chili Con Queso**

WEEK 4: Day 5

Breakfast: Spinach and Cheese Egg Bake**

Lunch: Beef and Veggie Noodle Soup ***

Dinner:

WEEK 4: Day 6

Breakfast: Egg Pockets **

Lunch: Bacon Wrapped Cheese and Jalapeno Stuffed Chicken Bites **

Dinner: Crispy Fried Chicken***

WEEK 4: Day 7

Breakfast: Eggie Cups **

Lunch: 'Everything in the Fridge' Salad**

Dinner: Spiced Moroccan Stuffed Peppers***

* Recipe can be found at www.wickedstuffed.com

** Recipe can be found at www.ketojourney.blogspot.com

*** Recipe can be found at http://nobunplease.com

RECIPES

A lot of readers asked me to put together a meal plan for more than three days so that there is a bigger choice of meals for you available. In this bonus chapter you will find ketogenic-friendly recipes that will benefit you and help you to achieve your goals. Enjoy!

Scrambled Eggs

What you need:

- 3 Large Eggs

- 1 Tablespoon of unsalted butter

- Coarse salt and freshly ground pepper

How to cook:

First use a fork to beat the eggs together. Then melt the butter in medium nonstick skillet over low heat. Next add egg mixture. After that, using a heatproof flexible spatula, gently pull the eggs to the center of the pan and let the liquid parts run out under the perimeter. Cook, continually moving eggs with the spatula, just until eggs are set, 1 1/2 to 3 minutes. Season with salt and pepper; serve hot.

Creamy Chocolate Milk

What you need (2 servings):

- 16 ounces unsweetened almond milk

- 1 packet artificial sweetener

- 4 ounces heavy cream

- 1 scoop whey isolate powder

- 1/2 cup crushed ice (optional: add if you like a thick drink, but the flavor will be less intense.)

How to cook:

Put all ingredients in blender and blend until smooth. This recipe can be doubled, as can most low carb smoothie recipes.

Fruits with low carbs

These serving sizes of fruit have only 5 grams of net carbs (carb minus the fiber).

- 1/2 cup of raw strawberries (3.3 net carbs)

- 1/2 cup of raw raspberries (4.2 net carbs)

- 1/2 of a medium peach (4.3 net carbs)

- 5 whole sweet cherries (5.1 net carbs)

- 1/2 of a kiwi fruit (4.3 net carbs)

- 1 medium apricot (3.2 net carbs)

- 1/2 medium Haas avocado (3.7 net carbs)

Protein Drinks

What you need:

- 16 ounces unsweetened almond milk

- 4 ounces heavy cream

- 2 scoops Whey Powder

- 1 tablespoon of Sugar Free White Chocolate syrup

- 1/2 cup crushed ice (optional: add if you like a thick drink, but the flavor will be less intense.)

How to cook:

Put all ingredients in a blender and blend until smooth.

Egg white spinach omelet

What you need:

- Egg whites (4-5)

- Egg yolk (1)

- Almond milk (2 tbs/30 ml) you can replace with soy milk, skim milk or coconut milk

- Tomato (half or 1 plum tomato)

- Shredded spinach (1 handful)

- Purple onion (1 tbs)

- Basil (1 pinch)

- Garlic (optional)

- Olive oil cooking spray

How to cook:

Chop the vegetables. Then beat the egg whites, the yolk and the almond milk. After that spray a small frying pan with oil and quick sauté the vegetables just until soft. Put the vegetables on the side, spray the pan again, put medium-low heat and pour the eggs. Cook until the eggs are firm, add the vegetables on one side and fold the other half over top. Add fruits to the plate and serve!

Chicken Salad

What you need:

- 1 large uncooked chicken breast, cut into 1 inch chunks

- 2 teaspoons Canadian Steak Seasoning (Tone's brand is good)

- 2 tablespoons butter

- 5 slices bacon

- Small tomato, seeded and cut into small chunks

- 2 ounces Muenster cheese, shredded

How to cook:

Sprinkle the chicken with the Canadian Steak seasoning, then saute it butter over medium heat until cooked through. Set aside to cool. Then cut the bacon strips crosswise into thin strips, and saute over medium high heat until crispy. Pour off excess grease, then drain the bacon on paper towels until cool.

Dressing:

- 2 tablespoons butter

- 1 raw, organic egg yolk, preferably from pastured chickens (makes for richer, tastier yolk)

- 2 ounces mayonnaise

- 2 teaspoons lemon juice

How to cook:

Place butter in small sauce pan, and melt over low heat. Do not let it get hot. Then remove the melted butter from heat and let cool (it should be warm, not hot). Add the egg yolk and whisk until the mixture is smooth and glossy. Then add the mayonnaise and whisk until smooth. Next add lemon juice and salt and whisk until smooth. Finally combine the salad ingredients and the dressing and mix well.

Portobello "Bun"

What you need:

- 2 Portobello Mushroom Caps

- 1/2 Tbsp. Organic Extra Virgin Coconut Oil

- 1 Garlic clove

- 1 Tsp. Oregano

- Pinch Salt

- Pinch Freshly Ground Black Pepper

Burger Patty

- 6 Oz. Organic, Grassfed Beef or Bison

- 1 Tbsp. Dijon Mustard

- 1 tsp. Salt

- 1 tsp. Freshly Ground Black Pepper

- 1/4 Cup Cheddar Cheese

How to cook:

Preheat your griddle to high. In a bowl, combine the coconut oil, garlic, oregano, salt and pepper. Then add portobello caps and let them marinade until ready to grill the meat. In a separate bowl, combine ground beef, dijon, salt, pepper, and cheese. Form the meat mixture into a rounded patty. Place "buns" on the grill and let them cook for about 8 minutes or until heated through. Then add the burger to the grill and cook for 5 minutes per side (medium rare). Remove the portobello caps and burger from the grill. Wrap that sweet burger between your two mushroom buns, and lay on the fixin's. Add sugar free ketchup, onion, arugula or tomato!

Turkey Avocado Rolls

What you need:

- 8 ounces cream cheese, softened to room temp

- 1 medium ripe Haas Avocado, scooped from shell, and cut into small cubes

- 1 tablespoon mayonnaise

- 1/4 teaspoon of granulated garlic or 1/2 teaspoon minced garlic clove

- 1/4 teaspoon onion powder or 2 ounces finely minced onion

- salt to taste

- 1 pound thinly sliced smoked turkey

How to cook:

Using a hand mixer, whip the cream cheese until smooth. Then add the remaining ingredients and whip about a minute more, until mixture is smooth. Next spread the turkey slices out on paper towels and pat dry if needed. Spread entire turkey slice with a thin layer of the avocado cheese mixture. Starting at one end, roll up the turkey slice like a jelly roll. Either you enjoy immediately, or store in a sealable container in the refrigerator.

Paleo egg muffin cups (6)

What you need:

- Eggs (6)

- Nitrate Free Shaved Turkey (6 slices)

- Sliced Spinach (½ cup)

- Red Pepper (3 tablespoons)

- Mozzarella Cheese Light

- Fresh Basil (optional)

- Red Onion (2 tablespoons, finely chopped)

- Salt & Pepper

How to cook:

Preheat the oven to 350°. Then slice the spinach, red onion, red pepper and basil and grate the mozzarella cheese. Spray a nonstick muffin tin with olive oil spray and drape the piece of turkey in one of the muffin cups. Now carefully crack an egg and pour it into the turkey cup. Next add a litte bit of sliced red onion, spinach, red pepper and cheese on top of the egg. Fresh basil, salt and pepper are optional. Put the muffin in the oven and bake until the eggs are set and the whites are opaque, about 10-15 minutes.

Coconut Shrimps and Avocados

What you need:

- Shrimps (1 cup)

- Organic peanut butter (½ tablespoon)

- Avocados (half)

- Lite coconut milk (1tbs)

- Sriracha hot sauce (as you wish)

- Coconut Shredded (1 teaspoon)

How to cook:

In a nonstick saute pan on medium temperature, spray with an olive oil sprayer. Then pour the coconut milk, the peanut butter and the Sriracha hot sauce. Add the shrimps and saute for about 3-4 minutes or until the shrimps are pink. Cut half an avocado in cubes and put it on a plate. Finally add the avocados on top and sprinkle with shredded coconut.

Keto Stir Fry

What you need (3 servings):

- Coconut Oil (1 tbs)

- Spanish Onion (1/2 medium)

- Brown Mushrooms (5 medium)

- Kale (2 leaves)

- Broccoli (1/2 cup)

- Red Pepper (1/2 medium)

- Ground Beef (300g)

- Chinese Five Spices (1 tbs)

- 1 tbs of Cayenne Pepper (1 tbs)

How to cook:

Chop the broccoli, the red pepper, the onion and the kale. Slice the mushrooms.

In a large skillet, heat the coconut oil on medium-high heat and add the onions for about 1 minute. Then add the rest of the vegetable and cook an additional 2 minutes stirring frequently. Next add the ground beef and the spices and cook for 2 minutes and reduce the heat to medium. Cover the skillet and let it cook until the beef is brown (about 5-10 minutes).

Mahi Mahi

What you need (1 Filet):

- Frozen Vegetables (1 cup)

- Hummus (2 tbs)

- Philadelphia Cheese (1 tsp)

- Lime (1 tbs)

- Coriander (fresh is better)

- Sea salt and ground pepper to taste

How to cook:

Place the vegetables on the bottom basket and the Mahi Mahi on the top basket. Add lime, cilantro, salt and pepper, basil or any other spice you like. Preset your steamer to 30 minutes. After the 30 minutes, put the filet on your plate, add the Philadelphia cheese on your vegetables (it will melt) and add hummus on the side.

SUCCESS TIPS

By now, you should have known what is a ketogenic diet, its advantages and disadvantages, what foods to eat and even a 4-week meal plan to help you start a ketogenic diet. However, all that information can become insignificant if you do not have the tips on how to maintain the diet. The following pointers will serve as cheat codes to help you get a grip of ketosis.

1. **Get a carb counter guide**

   In ketosis the carb count can determine if you succeed or fail. A carb counter guide will give you a list of foods and their carb or calorie values. This will enable you to pick foods that are low on calories to fit your diet.

2. **Clear out the carbs**

   If you want to start on a ketosis diet, it is probably best you clear your house of any high carb foods. This can range from your cereals to your fruits and even your sodas. This will make it easier for one not to revert from ketosis due to temptations and cravings.

3. **Restock your kitchen**

   After clearing the house of any high carb foods, restock the house with low carb diet foods. This will especially help in your ketogenic diet since it will make sure you are on low carb foods all the time weather it is snacks or regular meals.

4. A ketosis plan does not mean a special diet. There is no need to buy any low carb packaged foods, as it only requires real and whole foods in their natural state. The

only exceptions are artificial sweeteners, which are important in maintaining a low carb diet.

5. **Spend more time in the kitchen**

A ketogenic diet comes at a price. There are not many readymade low carb foods in the market; most have to be cooked. Therefore, if you do not like cooking, you had better start practicing if you are to achieve your set goals and targets.

6. **Think and plan your meals**

You have to really think and plan ahead of meals. This ensures that you buy the right foods from the store and helps you stick to your schedule. For example, if you know that you are having tuna and broccoli for dinner, having a good plan will eliminate chances of opting for high carb foods.

7. **Changing your habits**

There is no compromise on changing your habits if you start on a ketogenic diet. Therefore, if you used to stop at a nearby coffee shop or restaurant to have pie, it is about time you stopped and embraced a low carb pizza.

8. **Drink a lot of water**

When on ketosis, your kidneys will start to dump out water that has been held by the body due to high carb intake. This means you have to drink a lot of water to replace all that water that gets lost. In addition, ketons in the blood cause a diuretic effect that can make the body dehydrated; therefore, you need to consume a lot of water. Remember to take plenty of mineral supplements since they are also lost with the water.

9. **Avoid high carb foods**

Avoid foods especially the ones on the high carbs list. They will only serve to raise your blood sugar levels, which will reverse the ketosis process. It is important to make a commitment to yourself to avoid high carb foods if you plan to start a ketosis diet.

10. **Take natural supplements**

Ketogenic diets restrict you from eating high carb foods. The problem is that high carb foods are rich in micro nutrients, which you may be deficient of. To correct this, take plenty of supplements to get the vital vitamins and minerals that you miss.

11. **Track your ketosis levels**

You can do this by buying ketone reagent strips that will track your progress as the weeks go by. After about 3-4 weeks, your body should be well adapted to the ketosis diet and the strips should not test negative for ketones. If they do, it means that either you are not fully adapted or are not taking your ketosis diet seriously.

12. **Track your daily intake**

Keep a journal or a personal spreadsheet where you will record your daily food intake. This will help in keeping track of your carb count and list of foods you like and do not like. You can also tell when you go off track.

13. **Do not focus on your weight**

If your main aim is to lose weight, do not keep weighing yourself frequently. Weights can fluctuate over a certain range because of changes in water intake and absorption. Focus more on health benefits and long-term goals. Eventually, you will lose weight although this has to take time. Too much emphasis on weight can see you quit the ketogenic diet.

CONCLUSION

Ketogenic diets have huge benefits health wise and adapting a ketogenic diet can be a great way to improve your health.

This book has taught you everything you need to know, the 'dos and the don'ts' of how to make your life a 'keto' friendly lifestyle and we hope that by implementing this diet in your life, you won't have to sacrifice all of your favorite foods. Hooray, for 'keto' right? You don't have to starve yourself like some of the other dieting plans require!

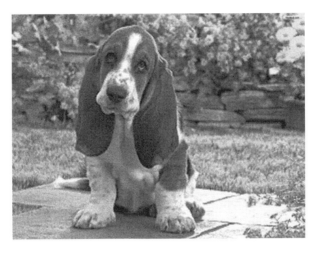

Finally, if you enjoyed this book, I would like to ask you for favor. Would you be so kind to leave a review on Amazon? It would be very much appreciated! Please review!

For any further questions, comments or ideas you can contact me at sarahjoybooks@gmail.com .

To your success,

Sarah

Preview of 'The Super Shred Diet'

If you are looking for an alternative to the Ketogenic Diet, maybe this one here is for you! The great thing about "The Super Shred Diet" is that you will have guaranteed sustainable results.

How many times have you ever started on a diet only to stop diet just a few days after starting out? I am sure you can relate with starting on a diet and stopping midway either because it was too restricting or just too damn expensive. However, dieting does not need to be boring, expensive and confusing. A good dieting program that can translate to a lifestyle diet should not leave you hungry and overwhelmed when you feel like you are doing something wrong if you do not follow it to the latter. If you are looking for a fast and effective way of losing weight and still enjoying yourself as you diet, then the super shred diet is just for you. While you may say that it is not healthy to lose a lot of weight within a short time, the thing is that the only reason that we have been taught that losing weight fast is unhealthy is due to the extreme and unorthodox methods used to lose weight quickly. You need to know that it is actually possible to lose weight in a healthy way. This does not mean that the super shred diet is easy, it is quite challenging. In any case how do you expect to lose a huge amount of pounds within four weeks when it has actually taken you several years to gain all that weight? Your body will thus need to be challenged to make it possible for you to lose that weight. Of great importance to note is that the super shred diet is a short-term program and thus may not be suitable as a lifestyle program. This program can however be a stepping-stone to better eating habits.

You may probably be wondering, what exactly is this super shred diet that can help me lose twenty pounds within four weeks? The super shred diet is a four week super-charged weight loss program. We will have a look at the principles that govern the super shred diet.

How Does The Super Shred Diet Work?

The super shred diet is founded on some basic principles that make it very effective. We will have a look at some of these principles to enable you know how exactly you will lose weight with the super shred diet.

Negative Energy Balance

This is one of the main principles of not only the super shred diet but every other diet. Energy balance simply refers to the relationship between the calories you get from food and drink and the calories you use when undertaking different activities during the day. Negative energy balance simply means that you consume fewer calories than what your body needs. The body gets its energy from carbohydrates, fats and proteins; therefore, when the body does not have enough energy, it will look for energy from fats to compensate for the negative energy balance. When we take in more calories than we need, the body stores the excess in form of fats. This means that when you take in fewer calories, the body will go to its reserves and burn the fats to get energy. The burning of fats then leads to weight loss.

The super shred diet has been specifically designed to create the negative energy balance. You will also need to exercise in order to create the need for energy, as this will then translate to your body burning fats to get the energy.

Calorie Disruption

This is the other important principle behind losing weight with the super shred diet. There has been a lot of research when it comes to calorie consumption, fasting and energy usage. Some studies indicate that intermittent fasting can actually lower your blood pressure. While the super shred diet does not focus on extreme fasting, you will experience a reduction in the calories you consume. For instance, you will be consuming a very low amount of calories in week three as compared to week 1 and 2. This form of calorie disruption is likely to yield the kind of results you want. The increase and reduction of calories is important in ensuring that your body achieves some sort of calorie disruption, which eventually leads to burning of fat for the body to get the extra calories thus achieving weight loss.

Sliding Nutrient Density

The goal of the super shred diet is to get the most nutrients from the least amount of calories. While nutrients from both plants and animals are suitable, plants remain the healthier choice. This diet is structured in such a way to ensure that you consume most of the animal nutrients in the beginning of the day while shifting to consumption of more of plant nutrients toward the end of the day.

Basic Super Shred Guidelines

In order to be successful and lose weight with the super shred diet, you need to follow some basic guidelines. We will have a look at some of these guidelines.

To read the full book, click here!

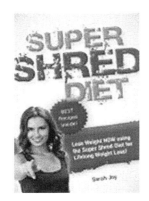

Check Out My Other Books

Below you'll find some of my other popular books that are popular on Amazon and Kindle as well. Simply click on the links below to check them out. Alternatively, you can visit my author page on Amazon to see other work done by me.

Essential Oils for Beginners

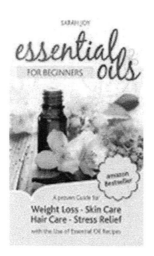

Top Essential Oil Recipes

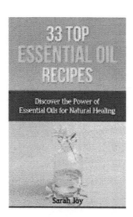

Homemade Body Butter

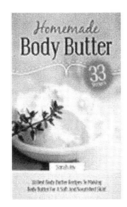

Reverse your Diabetes

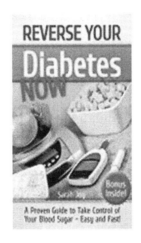

Cholesterol Solution

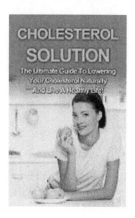

Blood Pressure Solution

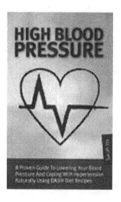

If the links do not work, for whatever reason, you can simply search for these titles on the Amazon website to find them.